"*This is amazing. Well written and congratulations. You are a wealth of knowledge.*"

Rachel Williams
Core Stability and Pilates Studio
Blackrock, Melbourne, Victoria, Australia

AF338228

Praise for **The Wisdom of Wellness (WOW)**

"David Grodski has a wealth of clinical experience and a holistic attitude to life and health. In his 2020 vision for health he brings both of these to bear on this easy-to-read and concise book covering 20 important health-related issues followed by easy-to-understand practical advice. A few changes you might make from reading this book could make a lot of difference to your life."

A/Prof. Craig Hassed, MBBS, FRACG, OAM
Author and Mindfulness Coordinator
Senior Lecturer at the Department of General Practice
Monash University, Clayton, Victoria, Australia

*"**The Wisdom of Wellness** represents the pearls of wisdom that can bring happiness and purpose to your life. These have been penned by a man who has seen into the lives of many people in his professional endeavours over numerous decades. Whilst it may be inappropriate to comment on how many years David Grodski has weathered on the planet, the fact is that he has the wisdom of many decades, and he has been paying attention as his experience and expertise have grown over the years. The beauty of this book is its simplicity. The key 20 points direct us all to areas that we can constantly tune and refine. It is a guide for life that alerts us to what we are doing well and areas that we may need to work on."*

Bill McTigue
Australian Sports Physiotherapist

"*This inspiring book arms you with the wisdom to transform your life regardless of your age, gender, or circumstance. It empowers you with knowledge and simple strategies to enhance your experience of health and wellbeing. David's holistic approach is incredibly refreshing, and I feel fortunate working with someone who moves through life focussed on living rather than just existing. I hope this book inspires you to do the same.*"

Meg Campbell
Holistic Health and Movement Coach

"*David's book is a much-needed resource in our modern times of extreme stress, burnout, and illness. His level-headed, clear, and simple approach is grounded in both clinical knowledge and a lifetime of personal experience, all wrapped up for us in easy-to-implement tips to invite into our lives immediately.*"

Olivia Downing
Psychologist, Coach, and Meditation Teacher
Livmindfully.com

"*What a wonderful book. You will help so many people with this – so uplifting and inspiring to read.*"

Rachael Downie
Success Mentor, Author, and Speaker

THE WISDOM OF WELLNESS (WOW)

MY 2020 VISION OF THE POSITIVE THINGS WE CAN DO TO CREATE WELLNESS

Dr. David Grodski

MMBS, Dip. Social Med (Ed.), FRACGP,
Dip. Landscape Tech. (Burnley)

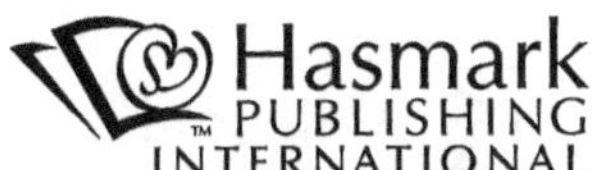

Published by
Hasmark Publishing
www.hasmarkpublishing.com

Copyright © 2020 Dr. David Grodski
First Edition

No part of this book may be reproduced or transmitted in any form or by any means, electronic or mechanical, including photocopying, recording or by any information storage and retrieval system, without written permission from the author, except for the inclusion of brief quotations in a review.

Disclaimer

This book is designed to provide information and motivation to our readers. It is sold with the understanding that the publisher is not engaged to render any type of psychological, legal, or any other kind of professional advice. The content of each article is the sole expression and opinion of its author, and not necessarily that of the publisher. No warranties or guarantees are expressed or implied by the publisher's choice to include any of the content in this volume. Neither the publisher nor the individual author(s) shall be liable for any physical, psychological, emotional, financial, or commercial damages, including, but not limited to, special, incidental, consequential or other damages. Our views and rights are the same: You are responsible for your own choices, actions, and results.

Permission should be addressed in writing to Dr. David Grodski at davidswow2020@mail.com

Editor: Kathryn Young
kathryn@hasmarkpublishing.com

Cover & Book Design: Anne Karklins
anne@hasmarkpublishing.com

ISBN 13: 978-1-989756-20-1
ISBN 10: 1989756204

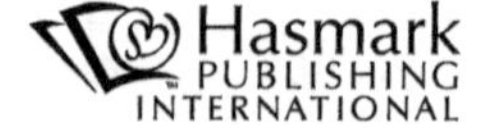

*To my wife, Helen, and
my children, Hali and Ben.
You are my mentors as you have
always walked the talk.*

ABOUT THE BOOK

The seed for this book was sewn in 1971 while I was studying Social and Preventive Medicine at Edinburgh University. The course was broad and covered epidemiology, the incidence and prevalence of disease, and how the management of morbidity and mortality was likely to be holistic. I also realised that the people who seek medical care sometimes don't need it, and those that need it often don't seek it. The stage was set for me to find a way to provide services to those that needed it the most. The course also covered the complex political and social issues involved in the delivery of medical services. One thing that became very clear to me was that to bring about innovation in health, one had to win the battle against the power of habit.

So almost fifty years later, the most iconic year in history – 2020 – has arrived. When I was young, 2020 was all about vision. So, in 2020 my vision is all about the Wisdom of Wellness (WOW). In this book, I have chosen twenty topics that can impact one's wellness and have given some basic background information on each topic. Each chapter also includes positive steps you can take to improve your wellbeing. I've added a sprinkle of humour to balance the serious side of life and to suggest that laughter makes good medicine. Each topic ends with a final relevant thought.

We all know people who do little to promote their health and others who get stressed whilst being bombarded with vast amounts of information and peer group pressure. All I know is that if you do nothing, then nothing happens or changes, and sometimes it gets worse like rust in a car.

So, imagine a red and yellow soccer card, with yellow on one side and red on the other. On the red side, you see listed the ten worst things you can do to impact your health negatively. On the yellow side you see the ten smartest things you can do to have wellness. So which side of the card do you want in life, which colour?

Will you be happy in a poker game with a pair of twos, or would you prefer a pair of aces? Remember, in life, you are the dealer. So get started in the wellness game and try lots of positive things to get the best cards.

You can find more information in larger books and from other authors who have brought together evidence-based ideas to advance the practice of holistic medicine. This book represents my personal views, and I have deliberately kept it small and simple. It is a manual for those seeking the least-travelled path and wanting to take the first step.

As Martin Luther King Jr. said:
*You don't have to see the whole staircase,
you just need to take the first step.*

So please enjoy my vision and remember:

*You only live once,
and if you get it right, once is enough.*
– Mae West

CONTENTS

CHAPTER 1

The Smartest Way to Start Each Day

Introduction

There are many ways to start each day. Some people start their day with a Berocca Vitamin B tablet, others with religious prayer or a jog around the block. Others engage with nature, experiencing the power of a sunrise or the exhilaration of a swim at the beach. Some might even stand quietly, breathing slowly and deeply, enjoying the energy of oxygenating their bodies to kick start their day. Whichever way you decide to start the day, please just promise yourself to make a gratitude list. You will never regret it. Never make an impediment list that has demands, control, criticism, frustration, anger, and stonewalling. A negative list creates chaos that can only be eradicated with sincere friendship, commitment, honour, and respect. Remember that for every minute you are angry, you lose sixty seconds of happiness.

In addition to a gratitude list is the need to have social interaction. We all need family and friends, but we forget to tell these special people that they are essential and important in our lives. We sometimes isolate ourselves and forget that friendship and conversation are available for us all. So, if you need conversation, make conversation, and if you need friends, make friends, and then experience the outcome of your efforts.

Remember, there are ten two-lettered words that make a profound sentence that can only improve your wellbeing.

If it is to be, it is up to me.

Positive Things I Do Each Day

When I wake up, I immediately write my gratitude list. This list reminds me of how lucky I am to be married to an amazing lady and have two children with dedicated partners, eight grandchildren, friends, hobbies, interests, and good health.

I have to stop and remind myself that the size of my gratitude list may be different from others and realise that for some people, they only have a small gratitude list or no list at all. For whatever the reasons, their list is a painful challenge to make.

But there are always some basic entries one can include on a gratitude list, such as having warmth and shelter, a few homegrown vegetables or herbs, and even some home-grown flowers to pick. The list could include the power of a sunrise or the colour of a beautiful blue sky, as nature is there for everyone. They may even have a caring doctor or neighbour or a pet that shows unconditional love. Sometimes people forget that 'somebuddy' loves them and they don't need to be alone.

Writing your gratitude list in a notebook can be more powerful than doing it mentally, so leave your notebook or diary on your bedside table and benefit from this very powerful action. This benefit has been scientifically validated as it primes the brain for seeing the good and overruns our negativity and bias.

The *second thing* I do each morning is promise myself that I will find a creative outcome (not just any outcome) to issues that may confront me during the day. I try to do this immediately when an issue appears so that I am not carrying any issue longer than I have to. I am then free and available for anything special that might come my way. How amazing would that be to feel true freedom? Sometimes an unwanted issue appears from nowhere and has three choices of action, but you don't like any of them. But one outcome is always better than the other two, and this outcome is the creative one, so pick it.

This technique of resolution was essential to survive in family practice, where I had to find creative outcomes quickly for each patient, clear my mind, and then totally be available for the next patient. I would repeat that process many times each day.

We have choices to resolve issues as they appear, or we can carry them for hours, days, weeks, months, years, or even a lifetime. By following this creative outcome suggestion you can be available and free for the next moment. This technique is very powerful, and once you understand it and practise it, your life will change forever. (Read the Problem Solving chapter for more detail.)

The *third thing* I remind myself of at the beginning of each day is the power of each moment. Each moment is unique and important, but it comes and goes. What would happen if we gave each and every moment our fullest attention? You may, I repeat, you may meet its need. In contrast, if you don't understand the power of each moment, you may have to be content with half-doing things, rescheduling, or missing the true nature and opportunity of each moment.

I then embark on each day's journey with gratitude, compassion, energy, and excitement. So be with each day and each moment and read the Time Management chapter for more details.

> *One day or day one – you decide,*
> *as this is a good day to be happy.*

Final Thought

START EACH DAY
WITH A GRATEFUL HEART
AND GET EXCITED ABOUT
THE GIFT OF LIFE.

CHAPTER 2

Nutrition

Introduction

Of the twenty topics in this book, nutrition is the foundation stone of wellness. Eating and digestion dominate a large part of each day. Unfortunately, there is so much information about nutrition, from so many well-intended people such as doctors, health professionals, and our dear mothers that it can make people confused. They all readily and authoritatively bombard us with their ideas, while magazines, TV, and the internet jump on board. Food labelling can take away our joy of shopping, while prepackaged food and home-delivered food companies wait in the shadows attempting to provide a worthwhile answer. This chapter on wellness will give you a basic understanding of what foods you should buy, eat, and digest.

Firstly, we have to delete those words from our vocabulary that want to measure everything, such as calories, kilojoules, diets, scales, and hours at the gym. Just say goodbye to them, as you don't need them. Why do we need to live our lives believing that the scales are always wrong or calories only give us energy?

So, let's go back to school and find two other words that will change your life forever. These words are not amazing, but their hidden message is amazing and will reveal all.

The two words are FLOWERLESS PAD. So let's have some fun.

F… stands for *freshness*. How lucky we are to live in a country that has so much fresh food available twenty-four hours a day from our markets, stores, and supermarkets. Other sources of fresh food are farmers' markets and homegrown vegetables, with the associated pleasure of gardening. Growing vegetables with children is even more rewarding.

L… stands for *local* and should discourage us from buying food from overseas. Fifty percent of the food consumed in Australia comes from overseas; what a joke! We can't be that precious to have to buy food from overseas out of season, such as cherries. Interestingly, only one-third of the food grown in Australia is eaten, another aspect of food wastage. Apparently, one-third of the food grown is not perfect, and therefore, does not get to the stores. Sometimes our food is outpriced by subsidised cheaper foods from overseas, which results in less local food being eaten and sometimes dumped. The other one-third expires in the fridge or is cooked, not eaten, and then thrown out. Surely we can do something about these wasted foods.

O... stands for *organic*, so buy organic foods whenever you can, especially chicken and meat. Shop around for the authentic organic producers. If you find them too expensive, then try to grow them yourself. Pesticide-free foods are preferred and are listed as the Clean Fifteen foods whilst the Dirty Dozen foods should be avoided. (You can look up these food lists online.) So eat foods closest to their natural state. There is a perceived belief that honey harvested from your local area can help with allergy and immune problems. Even in the Central Business District (CBD) of Melbourne, rooftop beehives are popping up everywhere. Besides these emerging sources of honey, there is nothing wrong with spreading your own body's sweetness – the 'Bee Kind' variety.

W… stands for *whole foods*, such as unprocessed grains, eggs, fish, beans, vegetables, nuts, and dairy. Why do we need to peel and waste nutritious parts of food, such as the skins of apples and pumpkins? Enjoy the whole food.

E… stands for *eating*. Try to eat in a quieter place, and always sitting down. The body is mindful and focussed without the distractions from computer screens and other electronics. The body's bloodstream can then focus on digestion rather than on muscles in action, demanding oxygenated blood when moving around whilst eating.

R… stands for *raw* and these foods are almost always better than cooked ones. An abundant choice makes food shopping exciting and meal preparation easier. So, with all the salads we are now encouraged to eat, will eating these salads ever become an Olympic sport, you may ask?

L… stands for *lumps,* so don't swallow any. This means you have to chew your food (mother's golden words) thoroughly to extract more nutrients and have your food adequately covered with saliva. Food covered in saliva takes the burden off the stomach and digestive system, promoting better gut health and immune system.

E… stands for *exciting.* Always plate your food elegantly to improve the dining experience. Foods of different colours, such as sliced avocado with sliced tomato and sliced salmon, always look attractive on a plate. This cephalic (visual, olfactory) phase of digestion amounts to approximately 30 percent of digestive capacity.

S… stands for *seasonal,* so try to eat foods in season, when they are abundant and often cheaper, in preference to foods that are artificially stored for months on end. By eating seasonal foods, we also can have greater diversity and receive a greater variety of vitamins and minerals over the year.

S… stands for *sugar,* public enemy number one when eaten in excess. We now have an epidemic of obesity, diabetes, hypertension, heart attacks, and strokes. My wife and I witnessed what happens to a community that changes from its local diet to a western one that has so many hidden sugars. If you find this observation hard to believe, then visit Bougainville or one of our indigenous communities. In Bougainville, we saw people in a country with no running water being sold fizzy drinks and beer.

Fast food shops were starting to appear and were now selling fried chicken and chips, whilst bakeries sold bread and cakes. With no supermarkets, little stores were starting to sell a few processed goods. Tea and coffee were being consumed with many teaspoons of sugar. Diabetes and hypertension were now common and communities with limited medical services are now struggling with these dietary changes. Now come back home and look at our society and see what excess sugars have done since the 1960s, the start of the obesity boom. How many more processed foods with additives and preservatives have appeared at supermarkets that can rob the body of vital minerals and add stress to our lives?

P… stands for *packaging*. Only buy foods that come in their own packaging and not a man-made one. Examples are avocado, blueberries, and carrots. Adhering to this idea would result in the removal of 70 percent of super-market products that are full of hidden sugar (up to thirty types – an alarming statistic).

A… stands for *amount*. Only eat the amount of food that will fit into the palm of your hand (roughly the size of your stomach) at any mealtime. Larger amounts of food only force the food already in your stomach into your small bowel before it is adequately prepared. Overeating can be related to stress on the digestive system, which can then cause many gastrointestinal disorders related to our fast-eating society.

D… stands for *drinks* which is the hardest of habits to change as most of us have always consumed fluids with our meals. When you think about it, drinks are going to dilute saliva and gastric juices. Saliva and gastric acid are produced more abundantly when the thought of eating or eating starts, so why would we dilute the digestive system? Ideally, drink an hour before or after meals and avoid soft drinks, which can have up to nine and a half teaspoons of sugar. Have at least two litres of quality water per day. Keeping one's fluids up helps the body to detox and feel hydrated. I hope one day that someone can explain why we need to drink water in a plastic bottle and often from overseas. The cost of fuel to ship it and deliver it is enormous. There is also an added cost of manufacturing plastic bottles, which are scattered throughout our environment and make an enormous impact on pollution. This problem can be seen with all of the plastic pieces and bottles washed up on beaches after a storm. It is okay to be seriously green with such issues.

Coming back to sugar, the World Health Organization (WHO) only recommends a daily intake of six teaspoons of sugar, but we are consuming up to three or four times that amount per day when you include hidden sugars. This has led to an enormous change in the prevalence and incidence of so many diseases that rarely were seen outside of textbooks when I was a young doctor. These changes can't be explained just by an ageing population, stress, chemicals, fertilisers, preservatives, or farming sprays. My common sense tells me that excess sugars (including hidden sugars) are to blame. Google the Cancer Council of Victoria website and see what they have to say about obesity and cancer, and then scroll through other information now available on the internet.

Positive Things to Do

- Throw out your scales or put them in the corner where the little liars should stay until they apologise. Also, scales can be misleading as they are not calibrated for heavier muscle tissue, fluid retention, or bone mass.

- Buy and eat real food. Don't eat foods your grandmother would not recognise.

- Plate your food elegantly to maximise the eating experience.

- Use ceramic or cast iron cookware in preference to aluminium or Teflon because of unknown chemical exposure.

- Drink at least two litres of quality water a day.

- Eat great herbs, such as parsley and coriander for their detox advantages; cumin and turmeric for their anti-inflammatory help.

- Select foods high in Vitamin B, such as whole grains, meat, fish, legumes, eggs, spinach, and broccoli. Choose foods high in magnesium to compensate for depleted magnesium in our soils, such as green leafy vegetables, avocado, bananas, legumes, and salmon.

- Organise frequent meals with the people you like including friends and children.

- Don't eat foods that have expiry dates on them as we will never know the true impact of preservatives on our health with the high consumption of processed foods.

- Preferably eat in a quiet place as this assists digestion. Did you know that prayer originally started at the beginning of a meal as it quietens you and allows blood flow back for digestion?

- Surely laughter helps digestion.

- *If it comes from a plant, eat it; if it was made in a plant, don't.* – Michael Pollan.

- Eat less sugar as you are probably sweet enough.

- Eat around the table, not around the TV.

- Try to leave the table a little hungry.

- If none of the above works for you, then write a letter to your stomach.

Dear Stomach,

I just wanted to apologise to you for

____.

From now on I promise to

____.

Love,
Me.

Let's hope you get a reply.

The good news is that we now have arrived where we can make one healthy choice from the above list, and then make another. So, if good nutrition is your goal or weight loss your aim or wellness your destiny, then follow any of the above advice and experience the domino effect.

You are what you eat, so don't be fast, cheap, easy, or fake. Ask yourself an important question: If you don't care about your body, where else are you going to live?

Final Thought

EAT REAL FOOD
AND BITE INTO LIFE.

CHAPTER 3

Supplements

Introduction

Are supplements essential for our wellness in a country that has such a wide variety of fresh food, fresh air, and quality water? There is a billion-dollar industry out there driving the need for supplements, while some chemists, doctors, and nutritionists are ready to look at possible benefits. Although there have been many studies done, few convince us of the need to consume vast quantities of supplements. I can appreciate that certain medical conditions, such as poor absorption in the bowel or certain chronic illnesses can lead to deficiencies. I can also accept that from time to time, people may want to top up untested levels. What is alarming to me is that there are so many people taking supplements who have never spoken to their doctor or health professional about any risks of excess consumption. The choice to take them is yours. I am not in favour.

Positive Things to Do

- Read the chapter on nutrition.
- Invest the money saved and buy yourself a good book or something special.
- Learn to grow the best organic vegetables at home.
- Donate a little of what you save to programs that feed the needy.
- Mentor your children about the power of consumerism.
- Get to like and respect the only real vitamin of life: Vitamin Me.
- Vitamin D is essential to those heavily clothed or who spend many hours indoors away from the sun.
- Vitamin B supplements may benefit those who are very stressed.

Final Thought

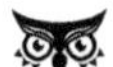

DON'T PRODUCE EXPENSIVE URINE.

CHAPTER 4

Activity/Exercise

Introduction

Everyone knows about the benefits of regular exercise. I prefer to call it activity (or movement) as some people perceive the word exercise (or sport) as an activity that gets you hot and sweaty. Or they find it competitive, where there are winners and losers, and so they turn away from it.

It is interesting that no other country in the world has a greater sense of recreational activity or relaxation than Australia. This can't be explained just by our good weather or the champions we have had. Feeling fit is great, but we also know how weak we can become by being inactive or bedridden. It only takes five days of inactivity for our muscles to start losing their strength and tone, creating dangers to our balance and mobility.

So, let's ask ourselves what joyful activity we could find to keep our muscle-tone and strength and then just do it. Some people like running, cycling, swimming, or going to the gym. Others like walking, Tai chi, Pilates, and yoga. The choice is yours. Remember, you can have fun when exercising.

A few years ago, while staying at Gwinganna Lifestyle and Wellness resort in southern Queensland, we were all reminded to be available for Tribal Dancing on Thursday. Each day we were reminded. On Thursday, we all entered this large room to be greeted by a very relaxed, creative dancer. As we stood in the room, music started, and we were asked to begin walking and weaving around the room and not to look at what other people were doing, let alone making eye contact. We were all just floating around the room, feeling free, and having fun. Before long, the music became faster and louder, and we were now weaving all over the room, flying our arms all over the place like young children. We were in the jungle. It was a wild and primitive experience. About forty minutes later, the music stopped, and we came to rest, realising that we just had a wild aerobic workout. We had had so much fun together. We then formed a circle until our shoulders were touching and stood there in silence, a very powerful, spiritual, and emotional moment. So, have as much fun as you can when exercising, even if people watching you think you are crazy, jumping in and out of puddles.

Sports psychologists and physiologists now favour interval training and strength training. These types of activities are preferred to the more vigorous activities that strain joints, muscles, and tendons. Although we were designed to run, especially from danger, we were not designed to run long distances and invite knee and hip surgery earlier than necessary.

Positive Things to Do

- Choose an activity that you like and not one that someone else has chosen.

- Do interval training for at least twenty minutes at a time, at least twice a week. Whatever activity you choose, do it for at least thirty seconds vigorously, and then have a recovery period of ninety seconds until the session finishes. This will significantly enhance your cardio-respiratory system.

- Do strength training with weights, Pilates, or yoga (selecting a comfortable level) at least three times per week for thirty to forty-five minutes.

- Drink lots of water when exercising to prevent dehydration. Drinks flavoured with mint leaves, cucumbers, or other herbs are preferable to cordials.

- Find other activities that come your way that can provide positive movement. For example, park your car at the furthermost point in the carpark at your supermarket and not near the entry door. Use stairs where appropriate instead of ramps and carry your shopping to the car in preference to using a trolley. Other opportunities for exercise abound at home when washing your car, bending and stretching whilst gardening, or doing home repairs. If you have a sedentary job, remember to get up every hour and stretch, squat, or go for a short walk if possible.

- Get off the bus two stops earlier as an alternative to an expensive gym membership.

- Remember to stretch before and after each dynamic or static activity.

- Don't let chewing be your favourite exercise.

- Don't get upset if progress is slow, as this is better than no progress.

- Accept that your willpower is a muscle – the more you use it, the stronger it gets.

Final Thought

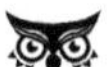

JUST DO IT NOW.

CHAPTER 5

Sleep

Introduction

Most of us sleep a third of each day. Some have trouble getting to sleep while others have broken sleep. It has become clear that no other determinant such as diet, exercise, and stress management comes close to having the same impact on health, healing, longevity, and function than restful sleep. As sleep is managed by the subconscious mind, we can't make ourselves go to sleep; we can only allow it to happen. That said, I am sure we can assist this process with the positive actions listed below.

Some people can bring their minds to rest between each of the day's activities. How lucky they are. Also, resting during the day has similar benefits to sleep at night. One of the great benefits of restful sleep is that it gives the body (liver, kidneys, gut, lungs, and skin) the optimal time to detox. Also, the resting body has the time to maximise its ability to produce its essential hormones. So, sleep and resting are not a waste of time.

Positive Things to Do

- Understand that if you have been physically or mentally active during the day, you can be more ready for sleep than others. So be active every day.

- Guard your sleep. It's valuable, and you need it. Don't allow others to deprive you of it. Don't let people or issues have free rent in your mind, especially when you want to go to sleep.

- Start any sleep rituals around 8:00 p.m. by turning off things like phones and computers.

- Finish your evening meal as early as possible.

- Avoid drinking after 7:00 p.m. to minimise disrupting your sleep with frequent trips to the bathroom.

- Ensure there is complete darkness where you sleep, even if you have to wear an eye mask.

- If you can't get to sleep, try shallow and deep breathing or count blinking. These are two activities we are not aware of unless we bring them to our attention. I find curling my toes will clear my mind of any distractions and allow me to go to sleep immediately. Repeat if necessary. Any of these techniques are more effective than counting sheep.

- My favourite sleep aid is to buy the best quality pillow on the market as you are going to spend eight hours with it. There is nothing wrong with indulging yourself in getting restful sleep. Get one today.

- The bedroom and bed need to feel warm and cosy for most people whilst others sleep better in a well-ventilated room. Try both ways and then decide the best way for you.

- Some people find soothing low-volume music beneficial.

- Have you ever seen young children drift off to sleep with unconditional love in their eyes when a parent sings to them or massages their back? Find an adult to do it for you.

- So now that you have the message, go to bed with satisfaction and wake up with determination.

Final Thought

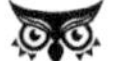

THE SHORTER YOUR SLEEP, THE SHORTER YOUR LIFE.

CHAPTER 6

Meditation/Mindfulness

Introduction

Meditation refers to the practice of calming the mind and finding inner stillness. It can also indicate the action of cultivating a new mind and emotional state, literally rewiring one's brain and body for good.

There are two common types of meditation. The first is called Transcendental Meditation (TM), which comes from the Vedic tradition and uses a mantra to settle you down naturally and ideally transcend thought. The other common meditation is called Mindfulness, and this type comes from the Buddhist tradition. Here one trains one's mind to be in the present moment giving positive attention to one's breath, senses, thoughts, and even emotions. You soon discover that behind all these happenings is pure awareness and the ability to be nonjudgmental and compassionate.

Not everyone finds these activities easy to do, and a simpler approach is preferred. While practised in some cultures for centuries, Yoga Nidra offers meditation and relaxation. This activity is becoming more popular in the West, as it creates a state of consciousness between waking and sleep. This yoga sleep is performed lying down, unlike the other two styles. Others try laughing meditation or follow religious styles of relaxation. Hearing ocean waves in real life or on a tape can be a simple strategy for relaxation.

I try another type of meditation where I instantly bring my mind to rest and have a clear mind. This exercise not only promotes my body's natural ability to detox, but I can do this meditation between each activity every day. This may be called power-napping by some people, but my exercise only lasts seconds or a few minutes. I sit in a chair or lie down and curl my toes firmly, which clears my mind immediately. If you need to curl your toes more than once, that is okay. This exercise can improve a feeling of vitality, prevent stress, and help jump-start productivity and alertness. Be patient, and try this exercise.

For some people, any meditation will be challenging as their mind is so full. Research from Harvard in 2010 tells us that 46 percent of people have other thoughts buzzing around in their minds while being involved with the task at hand (that is, their mind wanders).

So, do you want your mind to be MINDFUL (present, awake, and aware) or MIND FULL (distracted, distressed, and on autopilot)?

Positive Things to Do

- Try any of the above practices. Online programs for meditation are also available. My favourites are Deepak Chopra and Oprah Winfrey, who do great meditations preceded by an abundance of wisdom. These two remarkable people understand that meditation can improve your sleep, immune system, efficiency of oxygen use, and production of anti-ageing hormones. They also say meditation can lower blood pressure, cholesterol, anxiety, depression, insomnia, and stress hormones. Research has supported these physical benefits. It would be great if they are right.

- Connect with nature, with the energy of a sunrise or the beauty of a sunset to create a feeling of inner peace. Walking barefoot also creates a connectivity with the earth or sand as it brings those textures into your awareness.

- If all of the above isn't your go, be kind or compassionate to someone and feel the inner peace it will bring.

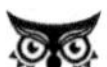

A WANDERING MIND IS AN UNHAPPY MIND.

CHAPTER 7

Time Management

Introduction

It is interesting that when you google questions about managing time, you find that each entry mainly talks about managing your time at work. No mention is given to the work done at home (almost as if it is unimportant) by all the domestic goddesses and gods. Also, managing your sleep time and the other hours outside of work are rarely discussed.

As we know, a list of tasks is useful in any workplace or at home, and being able to assess the importance and urgency of each task is helpful. Remember that sometimes a task may be important and needs to be done now versus later. Other times a task may be unimportant but still needs to be done now versus later. Either way, assess the value and importance of the task and move ahead with purpose and flexibility.

For most of us, each day involves rushing about pursuing careers, interests, hobbies, and fulfilling our responsibilities. We are busy, busy, and busy.

How often have we heard that if you want a job done, find a busy man or woman?

The reality is either you run the day or the day runs you. So, let's have some fun and move on.

Positive Things to Do

- This section looks at time management for the whole day. So, divide your day into three equal parts of eight hours. And guess what, three eights equals twenty-four (a mathematical equation that allows you to have your life in balance and harmony). You now have eight hours to sleep peacefully and restfully and eight hours to work passionately.

  And guess what? You now have eight hours left to be amazing. I mean amazing. My definition of being amazing is when whatever is important to you in your life is never put on rations. This idea is one of the most profound messages in this book. Another way of getting this great thought to you is explained by Jimmy John's motto: *The difference between ordinary and extraordinary is just that little extra.*

  So, if you want to be an amazing or extraordinary father, a musician, a good neighbour, or anything else, you must allocate enough time to maximise your choice. Usually, these choices or commitments to be amazing can take place after sleeping and working have been completed in the so-called third eight hours. Unfortunately, most of us lack structure in this third eight-hour period and therefore miss the opportunity to concentrate on a few important things in our life. I am not saying we waste our time; I am just saying it is better to do a few things really well instead of jumping on a horse and riding in all directions.

A new mother or someone with a new business can't have their life in balance as suggested above, but they can regain the balance when the time is right. An opportunity for balance for busy fathers, for example, is to pick their child up from school even if they have not done that before. Can you imagine the impact on your child or community if you picked your child up from school, even once a week during your working eight hours? Or, imagine the positive reaction you would create if you rang someone you love and just said, 'Hi, I have been thinking about you'. These actions can happen during any time of your day and can be performed whenever decided, and not in the so-called third eight-hour period. I am sure you can find specific moments of action during your busy day to acknowledge something or someone important that will create profound outcomes. As a doctor, I was constantly amazed at how often those people whose lives were in balance rarely came to see me. Sometimes I had to ask if I was still their doctor of choice, as I had not seen them for a long time. They would reaffirm that they rarely saw a doctor, and I really was their only doctor.

- In addition to understanding the three times eight formula, never forget the importance of each moment that you have, and always give it your fullest attention.

- Understand the power that if three eights really does equal twenty-four, then your life could have more harmony and balance.

- The secret to personal harmony is to delete all of life's distractions that are not important. Just open the window and let them fly out, leaving the window open long enough for something special to fly in.

Final Thought

BE AMAZING
FOR AT LEAST EIGHT HOURS
EACH DAY.

CHAPTER 8

Problem Solving

Introduction

Problems or challenges often appear from nowhere each day. Confronting these problems can cause stress and anxiety. Everyone tries with variable success to resolve these stresses and overcome a feeling of inadequacy and/or failure. All of us have wished we had hindsight or had handled a situation more creatively. Often when confronting a problem, we are only guided by two instincts: a situation of gain or a feeling of pain where others must be exposed or inflicted with our problems. Often these two instincts are performed subconsciously, and this lack of awareness creates the chaos that follows.

Some people, when challenged, are driven by the cortisol/adrenalin end of the scale and go straight to the blame, attack, and defend corner. Often they are unaware that cortisol production by the adrenal glands is the initial response (followed by adrenalin release) in the fight or flight reaction that was so necessary when we were threatened by wild animals and other life-threatening events. This fight or flight response seems to be of little value today, but one can't just reprogram our DNA inheritance and act calmly all the time. Others are fortunate as they are at the rest/digest end of the scale and want awareness, accountability, and understanding.

So, we have at least eleven choices when we are confronted with unwanted issues. Some of these choices offer less stress or no stress at all and will help you find creative outcomes (and not just any outcome).

Just try a few of the constructive choices below and enjoy the mental freedom they bring, remembering it is a good day to be happy.

Positive Things to Do (Choices You Have)

- If your *first choice* is to do nothing about a problem, you then own it. That is, you can carry it for hours, days, weeks, months, years, or even a lifetime. This is the worst choice. Remember, if you do nothing, nothing will change, or sometimes the problem may get worse. It is like seeing a rust spot on your car and doing nothing about it. Come back in a year and guess what has happened?

- A *second choice* is to overreact and become frustrated, irrational, angry, or even aggressive. This latter reaction is called rage. This is a common choice, and the TV has many segments each night about family violence, street fights, and neighbourly disputes that display this approach. Also, remember that the self-inflicted situation of stress occurs when you make a claim to do something that is not easy to accomplish. You may become frustrated, angry, and enraged. So always check on what claims you make in life and make them realistic and achievable.

- A *third choice* is to remain calm and explain to the other person that they will not gain anything if rage is their choice. This advice may seem like a trigger for further frustration for the other person, so just stay calm, and if you can, say, 'Thank you for explaining your position. I now know how you feel about this issue'. Not going into battle with someone helps defuse the situation and not polarise it. Avoid too much further discussion at this point. Repeat if necessary, 'I understand, I understand'. You now have created a situation for further communication and possible resolution, having saved the moment from disaster. I hope you can try this choice just once and find out how powerful it is.

- A *fourth choice* is to let things go when knowing they will probably not be so important the next day. Letting something go creates a feeling of freedom that allows you to be available for something special that may come your way. Why waste valuable time with unimportant issues when we are so time-poor. Remember, there is always a wicketkeeper, so step aside and let the nasty ball pass you by. You are allowed to sledge in this situation and say goodbye or condemn something unimportant.

- A *fifth choice*, which I like, is when you *seek good company and starve bad*. This choice may appear arrogant, but you can seriously minimise issues if you are not around people who are carrying their negativity and feel you need to be part of it. So spend time with people who will share their energy with you and not sap yours. Of course, as a doctor, identifying personal problems in patients and others and managing them is important, and the job does not warrant starving bad company. Let professional people manage those who feel negative. We do have choices, and we can plan to spend more time with people who we enjoy.

- A *sixth choice* is to learn how to find creative outcomes, every time, for any situation. Sometimes you have an issue, and you know why you have it. Sometimes there are several choices to minimise or solve the problem, but you do not like any of them. Try to find the best of these choices and take it, as this is the most creative one, and move on.

- I have never tried this *seventh choice*, but if you can make someone laugh when they are frustrated or angry, they will struggle to remain angry, and so you both could have a happier outcome.

- Compromise is the *eighth choice*, but I prefer either to let things go if they appear unimportant or preferably find the most creative outcome.

- A *ninth choice* is to learn relaxation techniques or learn how to practise slow and deep breathing. These two practices can lower raised cortisol and adrenalin levels.

- If none of the above works, then the *tenth choice* is to go for a walk to clear your mind by connecting with mother nature.

- The *eleventh choice* for some people is to exercise vigorously to deplete their adrenalin levels, which helps them settle down.

Decide which choice serves you the best as you may be the only person who knows the best path forward. Ideally, once you have made your choice, your cells might sing.

Final Thought

ONLY FIND CREATIVE OUTCOMES (AND NOT JUST ANY OUTCOME) TO PROBLEMS.

CHAPTER 9

Family Dynamics

Introduction

People have always said that there are only two families in the world, the haves and the have nots. I have found that every family is different, and they each handle difficult situations in their own unique way. Each modern family struggles to cope with the demands of modern life and the massive social changes that have occurred over the past seventy years.

Major changes have seen older people become institutionalised, more women entering the workforce, and the common dispersion of families when they decide to live interstate or overseas. These changes have led to the isolation of each family from its traditional support systems of the past. This isolation has been magnified when the concept and acceptance of community values and religion (with all of its wisdom and morals) have also changed. And so, the sources of mentors and family support structures have shrivelled up. Time-poor parents have to struggle on their own to allocate the time needed for everything in the home paddock to be at its best. Too often, families hold onto grievances and resentments as they strive to get ahead and now have to cope with these additional burdens.

Years ago, I witnessed a powerful program called Forum, where nearly 1500 people attended a continuous session over three days to learn the power of letting things go, but more importantly, to replace the past with a desirable future. The first two days allowed people to talk about their lives and grievances. Then, this exciting thing happened when we were all shown how to tackle our perceived burdens. I was surprised to see how many people held grievances against their fathers more than any other group. So, the facilitator invited us all to ring the person (even though it was late at night) who we thought we had the grievance with, and say, for example, 'Hi Dad, I just wanted you to know that if I held any grievance or resentment towards you in the past, I have now let it go'. Furthermore, 'Dad, in the future, I want to have a relationship with you that has love, integrity, and respect'. Some people had been carrying these grievances for a long time, even years, and found it challenging now to confront them. To my surprise, most people had a positive response, where the person on the other end of the phone stated that that was exactly what they wanted. A few people failed because of events beyond their control when people receiving the call were affected by alcohol or rejected the call as it was late at night. The facilitator calmly told those people to retry at a better moment.

Another family issue to contend with is lowered self-esteem in a family member. This issue does not necessarily come from being put down. It may come from never being told how well you did at this or that, or it may come from being uncertain about a direction to take. Whatever the reason, it is a terrible burden to have. A practical exercise you can do to enhance your self-esteem is to do a SWOT analysis. On a piece of paper, make four headings: STRENGTHS, WEAKNESSES, OPPORTUNITIES, and THREATS. Enter the appropriate details as known under each of the headings. You will be surprised by how many strengths you have. This is also a great exercise in business, buying a home, or assessing whatever.

So, what can we do to create family wellness that will bring lasting relationships that contribute to a meaningful life?

Positive Things You Can Do

- Read the sections in this book that discuss adolescence, time management, and problem-solving.

- Express appreciation and affection whenever you can.

- Experience and protect the power of the dinner table as an opportunity to enjoy each other's company and hear about any highs of that day and learn how they managed any lows.

- Be open, honest, and respectful.

- Believe in yourself and your judgment to create self-esteem, and then you can give every part of your life your best shot.

  Be who you are and say what you feel, because those who mind, don't matter, and those who matter, don't mind. – Dr. Seuss

- Learn more about yourself and the more fascinated you will become.

- Believe that you and your family are part of a team and so experience the benefits of doing things together.

- Learn how to find forgiveness and let things go.

- Respect that we are all different, and our passions, interests, hobbies, and anxieties all vary.

- Never give up; great things take time.

Final Thought

TO FIND FORGIVENESS IS TO FIND FREEDOM.

CHAPTER 10

Children/Adolescents

Introduction

The rearing of children is an exciting and demanding time, where you are on call twenty-four hours a day, seven days a week, for years ahead. There is no pay or super-annuation available and rarely an exclusive holiday with your partner. At birth, there is an overwhelming sense of responsibility and emotion and an awareness of no language for almost two years. How scary! Our daily routine involves feeding, bathing, dressing, and cuddling. Although smiles from babies are encouraging and gorgeous, there can be a feeling of inadequacy attempting to comprehend a baby's cry. Is it from hunger or is it in pain, or what?

With no previous experience prior to the first baby, these are moments of great concern that can reinforce the sense of inadequacy and responsibility. Were we expecting things to get easier? By the age of two, communication is the only thing that becomes easier as we soon find our child has entered the 'terrible twos' stage, followed by the so-called 'troublesome threes' stage, and the next year the 'frustrated fours' stage.

While working these natural stages out, and the full meaning of this twenty-four hour a day job, the 'fascinating fives' comes along to save the day. We have survived the miracle of birth and now watch our children grow and arrive at the new stage of adolescence (ten to nineteen-year-olds). A unique and even more challenging time awaits us.

Promoting the adolescent's psychological wellbeing is crucial, as they are constantly bombarded with desires of autonomy, peer group pressure, the internet, and old-fashioned parameters like family, cultural, religious, and community values. In the home, family unity is often only an ideal, and mentors are hard to find. Busy parents and financial imperatives complicate everything else. Evidence of eating and sleeping disorders and mental health determinants are aggravated by risk-taking behaviours of this inquisitive group. Furthermore, career planning and adult expectations challenge each adolescent. The pressures on our kids have led to a tragic increase in youth suicide.

Another pressure on children is related to the fact that our communities are run in a vertical model. In this model, children learn that I am your teacher, and you are my pupil. I am your employer, and you are my employee. I am your doctor, and you are my patient. And finally, I am your parent, and you are my child. This model always has someone coming second. What would happen if we thought horizontally, where we see the family as a team, and we move together in all directions as a football team does? This change of vertical versus horizontal thinking is an exciting opportunity for all families and can start as early as eight or nine years of age or possibly earlier. For example, ask your child respectfully what is their attitude to this or that in preference to telling them what to do all the time.

The other major change that impacts our ability to raise children easily is the dismantling of the old-fashioned family unit. When I was young, it was not uncommon to have a grandparent living in a bungalow in the rear garden. This person taught everyone at home how to grow this or that, how to preserve, and even how to repair everything. Also, my mother was a career mum, like every other mother in the street. We played on the streets with all the other kids and went home to our caring mothers, who also had the time to teach us so much about family and community values. Careers for both parents are equally important, but no one asked how we could replace these vital teachers at home. Around the corner, there was a sister or brother with their respective families and even an unmarried aunt. This extended family was unconditionally available to support their families when needed. How much has changed for the modern-day parents since the cavalry, as I called it, has bolted.

Fortunately, modern educationalists are aware of these dramatic social changes that can't be reversed and have introduced the power of positive education. We can now recognise many positive traits in children (such as creativity, curiosity, love of learning, courage, resilience, kindness, gratitude, and justice), which can be reinforced at school or in after-school activities. All children are born with some of these traits, while others can develop newer ones along the way. When you are time-poor, you may not be in the position to recognise these valuable traits, let alone reinforce them or encourage new ones. So, what does the modern parent do to harness these traits and focus on their child's reality and not a child's shortcomings?

To explain this line of thinking, what would happen if I gave you a sentence with approximately eleven words, such as 'You need four or five traits to live happily ever after' and I misspelled one word? You would probably say, 'This word is spelled incorrectly' and never say, 'Wow, this sentence has eleven words in it, and guess what, ten are spelled correctly'. Why do we always gravitate to the one thing that is not right? The answer to why we do this with our kids all the time is because our parents probably did it to us.

Furthermore, science tells us that this negativity bias we have as human beings was important for our species' survival, but now this bias aggravates the opportunity to think positively. We have never been shown the advantages of positive thinking that can make our children more resilient when they are not with us. Our job as human beings now is to upgrade our mental hardware and move our thinking forward.

Another factor impacting our children has been the power of social media and the effects of technology on their mental and physical health. We hear about cyberbullying and the negative impact on health with childhood inactivity and spending too many hours with their phones and toy games. How many parents going to bed at night are pleading for their child or children to turn that device off?

How can we find powerful things to say or do with our children, which I can guarantee will create an easier journey through childhood and adolescence?

Read on.

Positive Things to Do

- Firstly, we must start to resolve or at least manage any trauma, fears, and regrets we have had in our lives so we can make an active choice as to the way we want to parent our children.

- Actively listen to them always, making eye contact when you can.

- Stop thinking *vertically*. When the time comes, respect your child's opinion and start thinking *horizontally* where the family unit acts as a team. When the occasion arises, and you don't feel comfortable with their opinion, just tell them, 'I am not comfortable about this or that' in preference to saying 'Do this or that because I told you'. This approach leaves the conversation open for further discussion and possible resolution.

- Try to read to your children every day. This not only builds their skills in literacy, but it provides them an opportunity to connect with you in a calm way.

- Never shout at your children as this quickly undoes all your good work.

- Only focus on their strengths as this helps build resilience and self-confidence. I saw a dad tell his child off one day for his average backhand in tennis. 'But Dad, I did win the match.' 'Shut up', said the dad. 'Your backhand was terrible.'

- Pick your children up from school at least once a week if you have never done it before. This sets a great example to other time-poor parents and the community. It also lets the child know they are important in contrast to them feeling they always come second in your life. I am sure many workplaces would agree to trialling such a positive action, especially an action that creates love and harmony between parent and child, and which can only promote an employee's commitment to work when their private life is in balance. To be able to do this, you may have to start work earlier that day.

- Create an activity that is exclusive to each child if you can. Examples could include jogging, bike riding, fishing, growing some vegetables, table games, making a model plane, cooking, or even trips to the library where they are encouraged to select their choice of book. Guess what? On arriving home, they are more likely to read them, especially with you.

- Limit the use of iPhone, toy games, and TV.

- Be a role model for your children where you can help them navigate tougher issues.

- Find mentor figures outside of the home, at school, or from local sports teams. The concept that we need a village to raise a child has merit, as it can give children confidence and aspirations to create their own support network as they see all the villagers as their mentors.

- Cherish the dinner table and eat together and talk about the highs and lows of each day. Plan to have breakfast together each Saturday or Sunday. This simple suggestion creates special opportunities for every family member to enter into meaningful conversation and show gratitude and compassion to each other.

- Say something special to them at the right time, for example, 'I like you'. This is much more powerful than saying 'I love you', which they are likely to know already.

- Reassure them that any perceived mistakes they make are really learning opportunities. This approach is much better than them living in fear when you say, 'Only make a mistake once'. What would happen if we made the same mistake again?

- Avoid saying, 'You are smart' because a day will come when they can't sort something out easily, and they could get confused. It's better to say, 'You are a quick learner'.

- When they do something well, acknowledge it. Either say, 'You did it well and to the best of your ability' or as I prefer to say, simply, 'You did it'.

- Make sure they get plenty of sleep each night.

- Set reasonable boundaries with your children while having high expectations.

- Have fun with your kids even if you have to buy a joke book and have a joke night once a week. You can never have too much laughter.

- Let them know that there is zero tolerance for bullying at home or school.

- Explain that there are disciplinary rules and consequences, and hopefully, you will never have to enforce them, especially if you have followed the above suggestions.

- And finally, make sure they have perfect nutrition and get plenty of exercise.

So, a little joke about conception and parenting to finish may lighten the serious responsibility of being parents. Three ministers of different religions were discussing when life begins. The first said at conception, the second said at childbirth, and the third said when they leave home.

So please enjoy your children whilst they live with you.

75

Final Thought

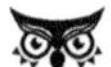

YOUR CHILDREN
COULD BE YOUR BEST FRIENDS.

CHAPTER 11

Marriage/Intimacy

Introduction

We all know that relationships at home and work can be challenging as there never exists a manual to help create desirable and workable relationships. I have observed that when a man gets married, he is thinking of his wife-to-be as perfect, and he hopes she will never change. Jokingly, we say that the wife-to-be is thinking of the needed changes ahead for her new husband. So, after opening the wedding presents, they realise that in the boxes of each of the electrical goods is a manual or brochure on how to use each appliance. They look at each other and wonder what are they to do without a plan or manual about marriage and intimacy and wonder where they can obtain one.

They soon realise that no one has been brave enough to write such a manual, and so they go down the road ahead playing a game in the morning and another game later that day. The game in the morning is called Expectations, and late in the afternoon, they play the other game called Disappointments. Many people become experts at this game and wonder why their marriage is so challenging. To create fondness, admiration, honour, respect, safety, happiness, resolution, and loyalty, one needs to follow the list of positive things to do listed below. By promoting these desirable attitudes, you may say they are more potent than love.

As far as sex is concerned, we all have our ideas. As Hugh Mackay (social researcher and best-selling author) has said, sex is the subject of more thought, more desire, more interest, more disappointment, more jealousy, more guilt, more time, more anguish, and more jokes than any other aspect of human behaviour.

Initially, sex was all about procreation in the early days of survival. Years ago, at the educational program called Forum that I mentioned earlier, the facilitator asked us all to remind him to talk to us about sex. He indicated that there was something profound to be said. After the fifth reminder, he said, 'When you are hot, you are hot, and when you are not hot, you are not hot'. We were all expecting much more detail and guidance as we sat there temporarily disappointed. We then realised that to create intimacy, one has to understand the true meaning of friendship, fondness, respect, and commitment to enable a deep and meaningful relationship to grow and enjoy its intimacy. To those who practise and promote these attributes, sometimes they believe they are more important than sex.

To many, monogamy has failed them as no manual ever existed. The traditional concept of marriage has now also changed, and those who have tried polygamy as an alternative have often experienced pain, anguish, and guilt for all those involved. Our attitudes to marriage have changed. In modern times, 62 percent of people now support gay marriage, whilst 82 percent of the population have become more tolerant and believe that consenting adults can do what they want behind closed doors.

So how can we make all relationships work?

Positive Things You Can Do

- Listen, talk, and share.

- Create a gratitude list of all that is special in your life and your partner's life.

- Never make an impediment list that has demands, controls, criticism, defends, and stonewalls. This list will break down any relationship rapidly, and I mean rapidly. This has to be one of the most powerful messages in this book. And if you decide to make one change in your life after reading this book, then don't make any impediment lists anywhere in your life.

- Learn to let go of the distractions of your partner's personality flaws and habits.

- Also, remember that letting go of a problem is more powerful than compromise, as you may not be able to change your partner.

- Find creative outcomes (not just any outcome) to all situations. See the chapter on problem-solving.

- Create regular rituals together such as eating together and holidaying together.

- Experience the power of intimacy in the inner sanctum of marriage, the bedroom, which is the one constant point of meeting.

- Guard your time together to avoid the pitfalls of not allocating enough time to something so important.

- A sprinkle of laughter is useful. We say humourously that it is possible that every conversation with your partner is to be recorded for training and quality purposes.

- Find your moral calendar (standards of behaviour, such as loyalty, honesty, integrity, tolerance, and humility).

- Avoid the power of habit. What would happen if every now and then you tried something new – a new restaurant, a new walk, or even a new coffee lounge?

- Understand that your partner may not be able to meet all your needs, such as your loneliness when they are at work, your spiritual needs, and some of your emotional needs. One does not need to feel insecure if someone else, or a sporting club, can provide what you realistically can't provide.

- Have fun whenever you can.

Final Thought

WHEN LOVE IS AROUND,
IT ONLY OFFERS
AND NEVER DEMANDS.

CHAPTER 12

Core Social Responsibility

Introduction

Do we have an ethical responsibility to act for the benefit of society at large? Can we have a core social responsibility (CSR) outside environmental initiatives, philanthropy, ethical business practice, and economic responsibilities? Ask the unpaid carers, service clubs like Rotary, caring neighbours, volunteers, religious groups, and dynamic personalities like community activist Les Twentyman and legendary people like Mother Teresa, and the answer will be a resounding 'Yes'.

Two years ago, my son-in-law, who is the owner of the Fruit Box, the major supplier of fresh fruit to the corporate world in Australia, was asked what his CSR was. And like most people, he had to ask, 'What is that?' After finding out its meaning, he and his wife decided to start the One

Box initiative by distributing enough food in a box for a family each week. These boxes containing fruit, vegetables, bread, and milk are provided free to those families with the greatest need. The contents of the box are perfect, fresh specimens and not recycled or retrieved products. With the help of local community agencies, families doing it tough around Australia can receive a weekly box of fresh food. In 2019 over 40,000 boxes were donated to families in need. Can you imagine the emotional impact on people when receiving something new and perfect in contrast to receiving something worthy but second-hand, such as clothes, books, and furniture? A bunch of celery in the One Box, for example, is sitting proudly on the top of the box and is firm and not limp. As you can imagine, receiving a One Box is emotionally exciting.

For me, I have been a member of the Rotary Club of Brighton for thirty-five years and witnessed the privilege of making other people's lives better, often through health and educational programs. A typical Rotary program can be local or overseas. It can be as simple as providing an individual with a book allowance, or it can be extraordinarily large, such as eradicating polio around the world.

Each of us has the ability and not necessarily the need to have our own CSR, but once you have one, your life changes forever. You may not be aware of the proven mental health benefits of helping others, but they are there.

Positive Things to Do (Creative Opportunities)

- Become a volunteer with a charity or service club, or even help out with a children's sports team.

- Do something local, such as a little bit of gardening or minor home repairs for a needy neighbour.

- Set up a free book exchange once a month with friends and share your old books to the wider community.

- Walk along a beach once a month and pick up any rubbish into a non-plastic bag and then bin it.

- Babysit, or granny sit, every so often for friends and family.

- Be ethical in all of your business dealings.

- Don't pollute the environment with plastic bottles. Bring drinks from home or buy one in a recyclable glass bottle.

- Compost your green waste when you can.

- Cook dinner for an elderly friend or a busy family.

- Reconnect with old friends – a card or letter is very personal.

- Become an advocate of your community (your village) and be the best neighbour you can be.

- Sprinkle compassion on others and your community to show them you care.

Final Thought

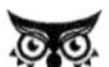

WHEN YOU GIVE, GIVE YOURSELF.

CHAPTER 13

Detoxing

Introduction

I am forever intrigued by the ability of the body to see, hear, speak, move, and think while behind the scenes there are these little factories making hormones, saliva, gastric juices, urine, and controls for reproductive cycles. How amazing is our genetic inheritance that determines hair colour, height, and gender amongst other physical features. These marvels of the human body, when combined, enable the body to have its own personality and to grow and repair itself as well as to cleanse itself.

This cleansing process we call detoxing, which helps eliminate harmful toxins from the body. What we do know is that the body has this profound ability, when healthy, to remove most of the toxins through the liver, kidneys, gut, skin, and lungs. In recent times, detox programs have become very popular, all assuming that your body can't do it properly itself. The most popular (but not necessarily the most healthy) ways to detox may involve the following: fasting, drinking vegetable juices, taking supplements or herbs, and using laxatives or colonic washouts.

Even though the available research is lacking, and often flawed, great results in feeling healthier have been experienced by some. These great results could well be attributed to the detox diets that promote eating real food and the advice given about drinking more water, getting more exercise and restful sleep, and limiting stress. I believe that we all have an amazing ability to detox naturally, and so the detox army that is on the move should be sent back to the barracks.

Positive Things to Do

- Read the section on nutrition.
- Drink at least two litres of water each day; filtered tap water is ideal.
- Guard your rest and sleep as you detox best during these restive states.
- Keep fit.
- Minimise known toxins such as coffee, alcohol, and sugar.
- Be proud of your body and respect your genetic inheritance.

- Focus more on yourself and listen to your body. Don't ignore its messages or suppress them. The way most of us live places additional stress on our bodies with inappropriate foods, lack of sleep and exercise, and exposure to environmental toxins.

Final Thought

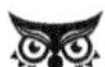

CHERISH THE FREEDOM TO BE YOURSELF.

CHAPTER 14

Weight Loss/Obesity

Introduction

Obesity rates have tripled since the 1960s. Weight loss is a complicated issue with genetic, social, and cultural forces creating the comfort most of us feel after eating. Consumerism and the availability of processed foods have altered our nutritional intake in favour of sugar. Food manufacturers have also worked out the bliss point for each product where the maximum amount of sugar is added to create the desired effect. Often this excess sugar is stored readily in the body as fat with the associated strain on our pancreas, musculoskeletal system, and our heart and arteries. The biochemical pathways from glucose (sugar) to fat are straight forward, as the body readily takes advantage of the excess calories and stores them for a rainy day.

What always fascinates me is how clever the body is by not releasing this store too efficiently, and keeping enough for a rainy day when sourced food is less readily available. This happens because the biochemical pathways from fat back to glucose are much more complicated. Often people who are releasing body fat have a decreased appetite due to the chemical process of ketosis (producing ketones), which suppresses appetite. So, what does this mean? Be patient when trying to lose weight as your body can't release its stores rapidly; and therefore, you can't see immediate results unless you starve yourself.

We can't be perfect, so just be better than you were yesterday. Just don't give up too early.

There are so many people giving advice about weight loss, and there are so many diets bombarding us that make us feel confused and abandoned. All the people offering well-intentioned advice require you to measure calories, kilojoules, weight, and hours of exercise. Overweight people sometimes have resorted to buying home-delivered meals, taking tablets, having surgery, and even trying meditation or hypnotherapy. Doctors, nutritionists, allied health professionals, and the slimming packaged food providers all have some success, but no one has the ideal answer.

So be prepared for some quirky advice.

Positive Things to Do

- Read the chapter in this book on nutrition for the smartest foods to buy and eat.

- If brave enough, have some visual therapy, and stand in front of a mirror naked for five minutes and look at yourself. Remember, if you cover up a problem, you don't have one; and therefore, you don't need to do anything about it.

- Work out the excess you are carrying as body fat and put that amount of kilograms (such as bags of flour) in a rucksack and walk around the block for thirty minutes. Stop and ask yourself how you feel. This little game can be life-changing. I once asked a patient to do a lot of walking (ten kilometres each day) to become fitter, and then ring me to tell me how he felt. He rang and told me he felt great, but he was 150 kilometres from home. So stay local in the beginning.

- Ignore fashion magazines and TV that only recognise one body type and just be yourself.

- Believe you are special anyway and see yourself as gorgeous. If you want to improve your body image, just smile.

- Drink as much water as you can to create a feeling of fullness and assist detoxing.

- Get involved in some regular exercise that brings you joy.

- Avoid harsh regimes that may leave you exhausted or break your spirit.

- Eat mindfully, chewing your food thoroughly and slowly.

- Do not ban foods unless they cause intolerances, as banning foods may set up a time when you will gorge them.

- Ask yourself if your current actions and thoughts will serve you or sabotage you.

I'm not telling you it is going to be easy; I'm telling you it will be worthwhile. – Art Williams

I am attracted to the keto diet above all others, especially the concept of having intermittent fasting each day by creating a large gap of time between meals. By having your evening meal earlier (6:00 p.m.–7:00 p.m.) and breakfast later (9:00 a.m.–10:00 a.m.), you can achieve a 14–16 hour gap. This mini-fasting gap accelerates the little factory that converts fat back to glucose, and so each day you do it produces outstanding results.

95

Final Thought

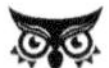

IF YOU WANT TO BE THINNER, YOU HAVE TO EAT LESS DINNER.

Good luck!

CHAPTER 15

Alcohol/Smoking

Introduction (Alcohol)

The consumption of alcohol in Australia is related to a powerful industry, a government happy to supplement its income through taxes on alcohol, and a way of life we all enjoy. The legal age for drinking alcohol in Australia is eighteen, while interestingly, in the USA, the legal age is twenty-one.

A close friend of mine makes me laugh when asked if he would like a drink at my house, and he answers, 'Yes, but lots'. The question then asked by us all is how much? As we know, the amount of alcohol consumed and its side effects vary from person to person. The side effects depend on their social norms, body weight, meals eaten, medication they are taking, the efficiency of their livers to process the alcohol, and their attitude to drinking and driving. Even though we are confronted each day with the downsides of excessive alcohol consumption (domestic and social violence, car accidents, and unseen medical reports), we do drink in excess. So, are there any benefits to consuming alcohol? Yes, it can relax some people in small doses, and this is good. It can also add to the dining experience if you drink with meals.

Even though there have been countless studies (without conclusion) on the acceptable quantity to drink, my common sense tells me the less, the better. Most advice recommends a maximum of two glasses (100 millilitres each) of wine per day or four light beers or one nip of spirits. These amounts taken at one time are a rough guide to a 0.05 blood alcohol reading, and so each person has to decide if the next drink is acceptable and when. Most of us have experienced at some stage in our life the downside of excess consumption, especially the next day. If you have felt that way, then probably you had too much for your body type the night before.

Positive Things to Do If You Drink Alcohol

- Drink a glass of water between each glass of alcohol.

- Don't drink and drive.

- Only buy your own drinks and don't accept drinks from strangers.

- Only drink where family or friends are around to care for you if needed.

- You can always leave a party earlier, so you don't drink as much that night.

- If excess alcohol consumption is impacting your health, job, or the social fabric, it is okay to seek professional help.

- Plan to have three alcohol-free days per week.

Final Thought

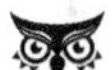

THE BEST DRINK IS FREE: FILTERED TAP WATER.

Introduction (Smoking)

Of all the things we should or should not do, smoking is by far the worst habit to take up. The tobacco companies have cleverly survived, knowing that addiction and medical hazards lie ahead. Also, we understand that every government has enormous income from the sale of tobacco products and is reluctant to lose it. Can you imagine how these two would rate in a morality exam? I can never understand how any government can derive so much income (often from people who can least afford it) from harmful activities such as smoking, alcohol consumption, and gambling. I am not a wowser who is opposed to alcohol; it's just a desire to see more moral leadership.

Let's get back to smoking and the impact of smoke. Can you imagine how our eyes would look if we still stood by our incinerators burning off household rubbish like we used to? Our eyes would be red and watery due to the inflammatory response to smoke. Well, imagine what the lining of our respiratory tract, especially our lungs, looks like after inhaling so many times with each cigarette. This congestion, which produces inflammatory fluid, disrupts our 'respiratory toilet' where tiny hairs sweep out any rubbish to be coughed up or swallowed. Like hairs on our arms when wet, they flatten out and lose their function. So, these respiratory hairs can't work correctly, and ultimately a chronic cough appears and eventually worsens. From there, we invite chronic bronchitis, cardiovascular disease, strokes, and lung cancer. On average, smokers die ten years earlier than nonsmokers.

Everyone knows how difficult it is to stop. Ask Quitline or Peter Mac Cancer Centre or every smoker.

Positive Things to Try If You Smoke

- In my practice, I had to find a way that gave people a simple and quirky way to stop smoking. So, as crazy as it sounds, I asked each smoker to promise to smoke their first cigarette each morning in front of a mirror. How crazy does that sound? But I did have more success than others, as most people could not do it. I was surprised at how many did stop. Once you can visualise a problem, you can take ownership of it and possibly create positive change. Nothing like a bit of the old-fashioned visual therapy.

- Seek professional help from Quitline, doctors, or hypnotherapists.

- Look at your family and ask yourself what role you can play in their future if you continue to smoke? Although this is an emotional approach, one is allowed to suggest this approach because we are dealing with a life-threatening issue.

- Try one of the great mindfulness resources available.

Final Thought

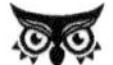

SMOKING IS A DYING HABIT.

CHAPTER 16

Ageing

Introduction

The increasing longevity of our population has created social, financial, and political issues. But let us remember that old age is a privilege not offered to everyone, and older folks should be happy about it.

An ageing population knows that birth is a beginning, death a destiny, and life a journey. What we don't know is how long the journey will be. We all fantasise that the journey should be long and that there should be some reward or recognition for making the journey and for getting there. In reality, changes can occur in our life as we get older that can't be seen as a reward, as these degenerative changes impact our physical, psychological, and social wellbeing. Diminished hearing and sight, reduced muscle tone, and strength are often accompanied by increased arthritic problems and fatigue. Your body is talking to you, often, and you need to listen to it. Although some human characteristics can improve as one becomes older, like wisdom and gratitude, for most of us, there is an awareness that changes have occurred, and these changes may even worsen.

Even though the exact causes of ageing are unknown, people want to ask what can be done to prevent, delay, and even treat our ageing bodies. There also is an army of people wanting to treat our grey hair, wrinkles, aching joints, and hearing loss (especially those over the age of seventy-five). Thank the humour in this world when one woman said she was proud of her wrinkles and wanted to keep them as she had earned every one of them.

Serious medical problems now appear more often with the outcomes of heart attacks and strokes, whilst cancer looms around for some. You would think these issues are enough, but dementia and the more serious Alzheimer's and Parkinson's Disease confront so many of us.

Yet we can overlook these challenges and remember that we are living now, where we can say yes to everything. In contrast, when we were working, we often had to say no to many important things in our life involving family, friends, and our own wellness. So, how lucky we are to experience those senior years.

So let's be positive about our senior years and embrace them with positivity and kindness.

Positive Things We Can Do

- You probably only need smaller amounts each meal.

- Drink at least two litres of water each day.

- Have adequate restful sleep and an afternoon nap if desired.

- Have regular exercise; for example, walking, gardening, bowls, stretching, and water aerobics.

- Make a gratitude list each day and be proud of who you are.

- Have regular check-ups, so health professionals can offer you the best outcomes if any problems appear.

- Find a caring doctor who is sympathetic to your ageing needs.

- Make sure you are not taking unnecessary medications and use pharmacy services such as dosette pillboxes for accurate tablet-taking.

- Check out available services from your Seniors card. Also, check what services your local council has such as transport, gardening, home nursing, and social activities.

- Declare your home as safe, especially in your bathroom and kitchen.

- Declutter your home using eBay and local charities that give to people in need close by.

- Pets are desirable as they offer company and unconditional love.

- Maintain an active social life with friends, family, and your community.

- If mental stimulus is required, then try University of the Third Age (U3A) online resources, crossword puzzles, bridge, books from your local library, and sudoku.

- Record your life's story or even write a book.

- Keep travelling and exploring for as long as you can to keep up with the grey army.

- Make sure your will is current. Try something powerful by giving with a warm hand and not a cold one.

- Try to keep your finances working for you as you don't need any stress if they are not.

- Start a new project like sorting out your photo album or teaching a grandchild a new skill. Try to create a sense of purpose each day, so you are part of something.

- Confront technology with the benefits of a computer or scanning new movies on Netflix.

- Be a role model for your family as you have so much to share with them.

- Have much fun and laughter with the people that are important to you.

- Don't wait for a health crisis to occur to realise how precious you are and what a gift life is. Change your life if it is necessary to support vitality, good health, and happiness now.

If you are getting older and need more care, then seek the best that is available. Don't live in the past as some people do when you hear them say, 'Remember the old days when I could do this or that'. Just be with today, as today is the beginning of the rest of your life.

Final Thought

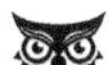

DON'T ACT YOUR AGE.

CHAPTER 17

Addictions

Introduction

This chapter of the book is the hardest one to write about because it is so complicated, and its worst manifestations can create tragic outcomes in life and impact the social fabric for all involved.

An addiction is a physical and psychological condition where an individual is unable to stop consuming a chemical, drug, or a negative social activity even though it can cause physical harm to themselves or others.

Sadly, addiction can also be tainted by criminal activity and erode personal finances with the government's desire to collect taxes on addictive activities such as cigarettes, alcohol, and gambling. Other commonly seen addictions involve the use of prescription and recreational drugs, shopping, eating in excess, and the use of phones and the internet. So, all these addictions cause health and social issues, and no one has the exact path to leave an addiction behind.

Maintaining wellness for those affected is challenging as they attempt not only to control the addiction, but they have to deal with any maintenance issues and recurrence.

Unfortunately, addiction involves reward pathways in the brain, which provide a rush of positive feeling, while the inquisitive young may tread where others fear to go, by ingesting an excess of a drug or doing something that has so much potential to create chaos. Surely peer group pressure is a major worry as well when people are initially exposed.

Positive Things to Do

- Make sure that they are eating real food, assuming there is any money left.

- Restful sleep (especially off the street) and exercise are also very important.

- Acknowledge that the addict may not see the problem and that their problem is not due to a lack of moral principles or willpower.

- Help them understand that it is not necessarily their fault that they have an addiction but let them know that it is their absolute responsibility.

- Let anyone affected know that treatments are available to give them some hope. Tell them your concerns and be positive. Remember, their mistakes are learning opportunities.

- Avoid using emotional appeals if you can.

- Find out about treatment resources like Quitline, Narcotics Anonymous, Alcoholics Anonymous, Smart Recovery, and your local or specialist doctor services.

- Remember that treatments may be individual or in combination and can include:

  - Medication
  - Detox programs
  - Residential programs
  - Psychotherapy
  - Motivational enhancement therapy
  - Meditation
  - Trauma therapy

- If you take excess prescription drugs, always check that they won't interact with each other and, more importantly, check to see if you still need them. It is not uncommon for doctors to repeat a prescription when patients request another, believing that they are not better or that they should just continue them anyway. Phone medicine in any form is dangerous.

- The pressures of social media and the big corporations have created an epidemic of addicted children and adolescents spending far too much time with their electronic toys. For children and others with an iPhone or internet addiction, try focusing on a balanced deal. Tell them they can use the device as much as they like as long as they spend the equivalent number of hours outside doing something physical or creative. For example, activities can include growing some vegetables of choice, jumping over puddles or into them, playing sporty activities, and exploring their gardens and local parks. Children can even have fun watching their chosen gum leaf going faster than their friend's in a stream of water. They can have fun finding flotsam and jetsam at the beach or garden bits and pieces, which can lead to an interesting macramé. Any outdoor activity also gives them a free Vitamin D boost.

- If obesity is a result of compulsive behaviour, then read the section on weight loss.

- Be available to look after a drug-affected friend, especially at a party or a music festival. You may save their life, especially if you have learnt CPR.

- I can't guarantee an outcome, but just try any of the above suggestions as they might help out.

Final Thought

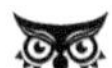

HELP IS AVAILABLE
24 HOURS EVERY DAY.

CHAPTER 18

Cancer

Introduction

I remain amazed at the apparent increase in the prevalence and incidence of so many cancers and autoimmune diseases. When I was a younger doctor, it was rare to see breast cancer in young women, let alone motor neurone disease, multiple sclerosis, and other neurological disorders. Most of these conditions were seen only in textbooks.

Although there have been extraordinary advances in the management of these problems, we have not reached that stage where prevention and cure are easily attainable. We are now living longer, but we are dying longer. There are so many more serious conditions happening in younger age groups now that challenge the medical research programs.

Unfortunately, cancer has a prominent position, as it has become the second leading cause of death in the world.

With cancer, there is an accumulated damage to genes that cause the development of abnormal cells that divide uncontrollably. Unbeknown to most of us, we are all producing abnormal cells each day, and we hope our immune system will recognise and destroy them. Every so often, an abnormal cell escapes detection and elimination, and so we have the beginning of cancer. Some people believe that stress, preservatives, toxins, and farming fertilisers and sprays play a part. Others believe that our age, habits, family history, and environment are equally important.

Recently, I have associated the underlying cause of so much more cancer with the changes in our modern diets, which has an absurd amount of hidden sugar. There are now at least thirty names for sugar used in processed foods to create the manufacturers' bliss point to make foods more desirable. This excess sugar (energy) is exactly what cancer cells need to proliferate. Even the Cancer Council of Victoria is commenting on the link between excess sugar intake, obesity, and cancer.

Additionally, cancer cells grow more rapidly in a more acidic environment, and so any substance that creates energy and acidity will promote cancer cell growth. Interestingly, our clever bodies can strictly maintain a blood pH of 7.35 to 7.45, which is slightly alkaline. Some people have moved to an alkaline diet to alkalize their blood pH against the threat of the acid-producing products when glucose is metabolised. The judges are out, but I recommend you 'watch this space'.

Positive Things to Do

- Reduce known risks by not smoking and minimise excess sun exposure and alcohol.

- Eat a healthy diet, exercise frequently, and have plenty of restful sleep.

- Maintain a healthy weight.

- Schedule an annual health screening and find a doctor who is inquisitive, especially if you present with a vague story or a change in your health. Detecting an early problem can allow your doctor a better chance of finding a more positive outcome for you.

- Support people with cancer by accompanying them through the cancer journey. You don't need to advise them, you don't even need to talk to them, you only need to be with them by surrounding them with love and compassion.

- Avoid stress.

- Leave something in your will for medical research programs.

Final Thought

WE CAN'T FORESEE OUR FUTURE AS THERE IS NO CRYSTAL BALL, EVEN THOUGH WE KNOW OUR DESTINY.

We need to enjoy each and every
day we have and remember:
*Yesterday is history, tomorrow is a mystery,
and today is a gift, and that is why
it is called the present.*

CHAPTER 19

Health Screening

Introduction

Many people have asked me how far and how often people should go in seeking early detection of disease by having early and regular health screening. Oncologists (cancer specialists) and cardiologists wish people had screening done as they often say they could have offered a better outcome if they had seen the patient earlier. Governments are often only concerned with the cost of health screening and not the financial savings to the community with early detection. Certain nasty cancers in the lungs or on the skin can often be prevented in most people by the cessation of smoking and the use of sunscreens.

I am possibly Australia's first medical postgraduate in Social and Preventive Medicine; and therefore, I should be able to give you some simple advice.

If you are willing to have your car serviced each year, with all of the obvious advantages, then why not have an annual check-up yourself. The type of yearly check-up needed varies with age, family history, personal habits, financials, cultural attitudes, and the different needs between the sexes.

It is worthwhile remembering that when you see a doctor, he or she only has three sources of information. The history taken, the examination, and results of any tests ordered. A lot of information is provided when a patient is allowed to give an accurate sequential history and is then adequately examined. These two sources of information, if performed accurately, can provide so much information that can result in fewer tests needed. The hardest thing for me to do as a doctor when seeking information was to have the ability to totally clear my mind between each patient and then be totally available for the next patient. I had to do this many times each day.

Another challenging thing to do as a doctor was to ask a patient as they were leaving the consulting room whether there was anything else that was important that they wanted to talk about. This question sounds ridiculous considering the ever-present time restraints that doctors have. Every now and then, a patient would reveal a crucial piece of information. Sometimes a patient would say, 'Yes, I have another problem that I have not been brave enough to talk about before'. Wow! The doctor now knows there is more than one problem, and the patient's history is not just a jumble of thoughts. He can't recall this patient back in because of his appointment system, but he can ask the patient either to wait until the end of the consulting session or reschedule for another time.

I never had anyone complain about this approach, as they were thankful that someone would be available for all their needs. Not all medical conditions that are apparent in the medical rooms need medical testing, and yet other conditions appear as they are leaving. This still makes us all vulnerable in not being aware of any early detectable disease or other wellbeing issues.

So, think of yourself in a decade of life, such as 40 to 50 years old, and realise how smart it would be to have some basic screening appropriate for your age. You may also realise that your screening needs will be different from someone in another decade of life.

So, my advice on health screening has to be general, as this book can't give excessive detail.

Positive Things to Do

- Find a doctor with caring skills, communication skills, and who ideally is inquisitive. Also, find a doctor who does routine tests in his rooms such as cervical Pap smears, urine analysis, and blood pressure checks.

- Have annual check-ups. At least have an annual full blood examination that includes a fasting blood glucose test (for diabetes), liver and kidney function tests, and an ESR test, which can indicate hidden pathology such as an infection, early cancer, or auto-immune disease. Tests that are useful as base readings, but may not be needed annually, include an initial chest X-ray, a PSA (for prostate in men), mammogram, and an ECG.

- Find a doctor who is capable of managing personal and mental health issues.

- Remember to give any doctor or specialist a better chance of early detection by giving them accurate and sequential information.

- Always remember that you are more important than your car. So if your car has at least one or more check-ups per year, then why can't you?

Anything that costs you your health is too expensive. You never want to be sick and tired of being sick and tired.

Final Thought

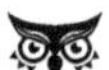

HAVE AN ANNUAL SCREENING ACCORDING TO YOUR DECADE OF LIFE.

CHAPTER 20

Finances

Introduction

Financial stress and strains can significantly impact one's wellbeing. Few of us can plan a budget, do our tax returns easily, have an emergency fund in place, or know how to plan for the future.

Positive Advice

- Buy a book called *The Barefoot Investor* by Scott Pape. He is Australia's most trusted independent finance expert. Read his new book for kids. He tackles credit card issues, insurance, and creating emergency funds, for example. It is also fun to read.

- If you have funds to invest and/or need superannuation advice, then find a local firm where your investment is likely to stay in this country. Banks and the financial industry have left a lot to be desired about financial planning, and so we are all left confused trying to select a financial planner amongst the so-called experts. Try to find an excellent firm of advisers that have integrity and who are more motivated about keeping and enlarging your assets than their cash flow.

- Be charitable with your assets as it is a powerful activity, especially when sprinkled with compassion.

- If enlarging your asset base and challenging yourself are important, then read the vast number of books by the financial gurus. These mentors will encourage you to have a good self-image, provide more service, work on the business rather than in it, and speak to people who are successful.

I used to tell my staff that in the earlier days, business was often about *I win, you lose.* This approach never worked, and people then tried *I win, you win.* I asked my staff to try *You win, I win* with clients and guess what? The business thrived. This happened because we focussed on the best outcome for the client and not on what money we could receive.

Great financial rewards can occur in business, and these are great when your life is in balance, and you know when to stop. The following story can remind us all of the merry go round of life.

A businessman wanted to retire at the age of forty with lots of money and live in a small Mexican fishing village. Here he could relax, write a book, catch a few fish, and live happily ever after. After a while, he could not help himself and went down to the marina to talk to the fishermen. He told them that if they got up an hour earlier, they would catch more fish and soon have a fleet. He was also confident that they would eventually have their own fish processing plant. They asked what would happen next. The businessman said you will make a lot of money. They asked what would happen then. The businessman finally said to them all that they could retire earlier and then live in some small fishing village.

Some people believe that money, more material goods, and status can bring them power and happiness. Others feel that the real rewards in life come from friendship, love, trust, creativity, truth, service, compassion, joy, and the appreciation of nature. You can make the choice.

As consumerism has impacted us all with the idea that we will be happier if we have this or that, our ability to find the ideal work/lifestyle balance becomes harder. Reread the chapter on time management and be in control of your life.

Final Thought

MONEY CAN'T BUY YOU LOVE AND HAPPINESS.

THE END

No, this is the beginning (of the rest of your life as your future is not yet written).

My vision is always to be amazing.

After reading my book and regardless of any changes made or not made, be proud of yourself. As Oscar Wilde said: *Just be yourself, as everyone else is already taken.*

IF YOU LOOK AT WHAT
YOU HAVE IN LIFE,
YOU'LL ALWAYS HAVE MORE.
IF YOU LOOK AT WHAT
YOU DON'T HAVE IN LIFE,
YOU'LL NEVER HAVE ENOUGH.

– Oprah Winfrey

ABOUT THE AUTHOR

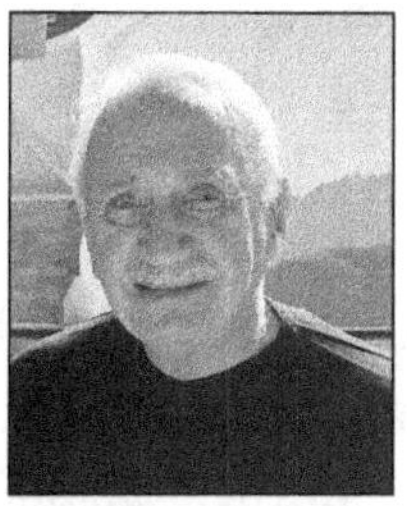

David Grodski is a retired family doctor who practised in the Bayside suburb of Brighton, Melbourne, Victoria, Australia. He graduated in 1968 from Monash University with a career path as a generalist, either as a physician or family doctor. His interest in wellness began the same year when a new chair of Social and Preventive Medicine started at the Alfred Hospital as he was finishing his undergraduate studies. At the time, the teaching of medicine was biased towards pathology and psychiatry, and little emphasis was given to other factors that could influence wellbeing, such as nutrition, exercise, sleep, obesity, gut health, meditation, personal finance, employment, family dynamics, and the impact of people one chose to work or live with.

After finishing his residency, David travelled to London to meet his wife-to-be, Helen. While waiting for Helen to arrive, he enrolled in a postgraduate course at Edinburgh University in Social and Preventive Medicine, which focused on a holistic approach in the delivery of medical services. On returning to Australia, he decided against an academic career and went into general practice where he had the privilege to practise obstetrics, paediatrics, and general medicine while providing a holistic approach for his patients. He also served as the Medical Director of the Brighton Community Care Centre for many years, funded out of Southern Memorial Hospital, Caulfield. This centre provided a complete range of paramedical services that were often carried out in people's homes, displaying the power of an integrated approach outside of his practice.

David's earlier life was influenced by trips to India. These trips showed him an enormous contrast to his privileged life in Australia and the immense challenge of caring for larger populations.

Later, he studied Practical Philosophy at the Melbourne School of Philosophy for three years, where he learned about awareness, being in the moment, human relationships, and the energy needed to be compassionate.

Thirty-five years as a member of the Rotary Club of Brighton has made him realise the power of making other people's lives better through health and educational programs.

His love of nature later led to a career in horticulture, where he has spent the last thirty years as a qualified garden designer and landscaper. His gardens varied in style but looked good in all seasons, were low in maintenance, and were reliable. He ran this career through his nursery in

Brighton, which he and Helen started in 1988. In 2004, 2005, and 2006, the nursery won Victoria's Best Garden Centre.

Two trips to Gwinganna Lifestyle and Wellness resort in southern Queensland were life-changing for David, as the staff confirmed that knowledge about wellness is much more available now.

He has also been inspired by mentor figures, such as Deepak Chopra and Oprah Winfrey, whose meditations offer not only inner peace but also an abundance of wisdom.

Finally, a fifty-year marriage to Helen (his most exceptional mentor) and his two children, together with their amazing partners and his eight grandchildren, make David feel very blessed.

He has learned a lot about life along the way and acknowledges that everyone has been his teacher.

He is possibly Australia's first medical post-graduate in Social and Preventive Medicine, and he is now ready to share his **Wisdom of Wellness (WOW)** philosophy.

The Wisdom of Wellness

supports

The One Box in Australia,
which provides
free, fresh food relief with dignity.

wwwtheonebox.org.au

____

A portion of the proceeds from the sales of

The Wisdom of Wellness

will go to

HEARTS to be HEARD
giving a voice to heart-felt creativity
for those who otherwise would not be heard.

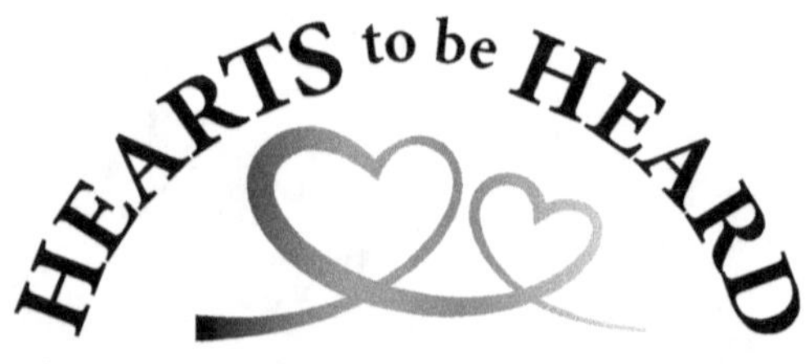

With every donation, a voice will be given to
the creativity that lies within the hearts of
our children living with diverse challenges.

By making this difference, children that may
not have been given the opportunity to have their
Heart Heard will have the freedom to create
beautiful works of art and musical creations.

Donate by visiting

HeartstobeHeard.com

We thank you.

www.ingramcontent.com/pod-product-compliance
Lightning Source LLC
Chambersburg PA
CBHW051808050726
47598CB00006B/2475